Rock Climbing

Mastering Basic Climbing Techniques, Skills & Developing the Climbing Warrior's Mindset

D1533094

Table Of Contents

Introduction

I want to thank you and congratulate you for purchasing the book, *"Rock Climbing: Mastering Basic Climbing Techniques, Skills & Developing the Climbing Warrior's Mindset"*.

This book contains proven steps and strategies on how you, as a beginner, can master climbing skills and techniques as well as how you can push yourself to improvement by creating the right kind of thinking.

We are born with an innate skill to climb. It comes naturally to humans like walking and running. We lose the natural ability along the way as we are told as kids that climbing is dangerous. We were taught that the consequences of climbing will lead to physical injury. So we climb no more and stick to pavements where it is much safer.

So how do we get that natural ability to climb back?

The answer is much simpler than you think. We have to learn how to use our bodies properly. As we face unfamiliar terrain, fear may get to us. But if we let go of fear, move our hands and feet over slopes and stones, we re-discover our sense of adventure. We reclaim our natural instinct for climbing back.

That is essentially what this book is all about. It is about learning and re-learning. It's about discover and re-discovery of joy, of movement, of focus, of one's sense of adventure, of being free from distraction, of focusing, of reaching the top!

Are you ready to climb? Are you excited? You should be!

Thanks again for purchasing this book, I hope you enjoy it!

Chapter 1 – Climbing is Movement!

To be able to climb, you have to move properly. Climbing after all, is about moving your body over stone. It is important that you find your balance with both your hands and feet.

Climbing is about movement. We have to understand the body's machinery. We have to learn how it works and how we can use it best for climbing. As we face more stones and slopes, we discover our strengths and weaknesses. We eventually learn to adapt. We learn how to make up for our shortcomings. We learn how to be in control, how to be strong. We learn to go with the flow, to move with grace and joy.

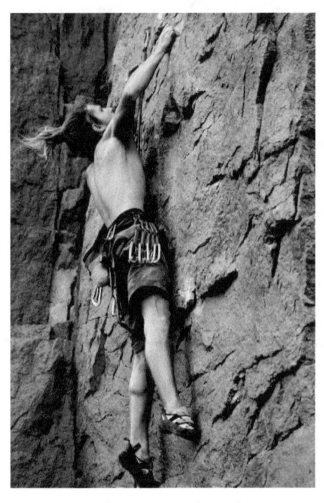

For many people, the first thing that comes to mind when they hear about rock climbing are safety gear and equipment. Of course, there is nothing wrong with thinking of safety first. Gravity is a reality after all. We do have to think about falling and its consequences. However, the essence of climbing has nothing to do with specialized equipments. Rather, it all boils down to movement.

This is why our first lesson has to do with ability. We start with the basics and the basics involve movement of our hands and feet. Climbing equipments are only secondary concerns but are equally essential to back us up through our ascent. So let's get on with it.

6 Essential Climbing Tips

We will begin with general climbing tips. Keep these general guidelines in mind. They will help you achieve smooth transitions and climb more efficiently and safely.

Look and Think before you Move

You have to bear in mind that climbing requires mental involvement as much as it is physical. Before you get on with it, take a good look at the rock surface. Take your time in studying the cliff face. Locate footholds and handholds. Find places where you can rest.

Do you see any chalk marks? These are what other climbers before you have used. Look for scuff marks and footholds as well. It is important that you think about your route before you make an attempt on the rock. Figure out the best strategy for climbing up.

Effort and energy can be easily wasted. Do not just rely on your physical strength. Rather, you must save as much energy as you can by using your head. Most importantly, you should stay calm. Remain centered. This is the best way to find a solution to any kind of problems.

Avoid hugging the rock.

So you love rock climbing, huh? It doesn't mean you should hug it out. Hugging the rock is one of the most common mistakes that beginners make. Remember, there is no need to get that close. Avoid leaning into the surface of the rock. Why is this wrong? You see, climbing is about movement and finding your balance. When you hug the rock, weight shifts from your feet to your arms. It makes it much more difficult for you to maintain your balance.

For balance, your body should be positioned around 90 degrees against the earth's surface. Your hips should be centered at all times with your feet firmly planted on footholds for stability. The movements of your hands and feet should be in sync with the basic goal of ascending but at the same time, keeping you in balance.

Rely on your feet.

Upper body strength is of course essential for any climbers. It doesn't mean however that you should only rely on them. As a matter of fact, you should use your legs and feet to push you up. Stand on footholds and push your body up rather than pulling your weight up with your hands and arms. Remember, you need to save your upper body strength for overhanging and vertical routes so whenever you can, use the muscles on your legs and feet.

Apply the 3 basic foot positions.

There are 3 basic foot positions you should learn. These are toeing, edging and smearing. Toeing as the name itself implies, is the use of the toes to grip on the foothold. Edging on the other hand, is about using both the inner and outer edges of your shoe.

Finally, smearing is about placing as much as you can of your foot on the rock. Take advantage of friction and use it wisely to keep your foot into place. You will learn more about this later as we delve deeper into foot work.

Keep on the rock with your hands.

While your legs and feet should be used for pushing and propelling, your hands and arms should be used for assessing and pulling on different types of handholds. In other words, you hands and feet should work in harmony. You will encounter various kinds of handholds. Use your hands to assess the rock surface with the goal of finding and using the best handholds.

Use your hands to grab and grip. Remember, you should focus on finding the best, not the perfect ones. Otherwise, you will be on the rock forever.

Avoid gripping too tightly. Over-gripping takes a huge amount of strength. It will eventually weaken you. When you are weakened, you are likely to fall off. As much as possible, you should grab the handholds loosely. Don't worry, you will learn more about handholds and finger grips later.

Move with the flow!

Again, rock climbing has to do with flow and movement. As such, you should avoid climbing in a jerky manner. Treat it like a vertical dance. The key to finding balance is grace. One movement should lead to another. Let the movements flow smoothly. Smooth transitions are essential.

Reach for the grip and grab. Step on the foothold and push your body up. Maintain proper breathing. Relax. Take advantage of big handholds and footholds so you can rest. Take the time to shake your arms and hands to keep the blood flowing. Keep in mind, it's a dance and you should be one with the rock!

Chapter 2 – Move Your Feet!

Our arms alone are not meant for holding weight and keeping us balanced. Our legs and arms together are meant to do that job. As a climber, you should work just as hard as learning the basics of a good footwork. Sadly, most climbers focus too much on handwork that they completely ignore the importance of their legs.

We've talked about keeping balance and using your feet. But how exactly do you maximize the weight rested on your legs and feet?

-Look for the best footholds.

-Position your feet in a precise manner on these footholds.

-Plant your feet firmly and steadily as you make an effort to move your body.

-Rest your weight over your feet and maintain a good body position.

-Practice smooth weight transfers between the legs and feet as you make your ascend.

-Always keep calm and stay relaxed.

Do you know why some climbers move awkwardly and tire out easily? It's because they focus on their hands while forgetting about their feet entirely. So here are some pointers to help you maximize the usefulness of your feet as you make your ascent.

Know your shoes.

Before anything else, it is important that you are properly oriented with your shoes. Take a look at the image below for your reference.

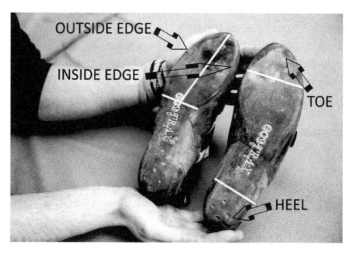

Image Source:
http://outdoors.stackexchange.com/questions/65
70/what-are-common-rock-climbing-footwork-
mistakes-and-how-i-can-spot-them

Which parts of the shoes you use depend on the rock surface's orientation as well as the shape and size of the foothold. In some cases, you may need to rely on the toe. In others, using the inside edge may be more appropriate. The most important thing is that you know you can depend on your shoes to get a grip on the foothold. We'll get into details about choosing proper climbing shoes later.

Move your legs up not sideways.

You will find out soon enough that there is no such thing as a perfect foothold. You have to make do with what you are given. But how do you know which one is the best? It's different for every situation but one of the most basic rules is to take footholds that are in front of your body.

Choose a foothold from shin to knee as much as possible. Avoid those that are way off to your side except when you are stemming or liebacking. By placing your feet in front of your body, you give yourself the opportunity to rest your weight on them.

In addition, you should also take small steps at a time. Don't pressure yourself into taking big steps. It will only take a toll on your body.

Avoid dirt covered rock patches.

If you see the hold is covered in lichen or dirt, clear it out first before you step on it. Before you make a climb, you are also advised to wipe gravel and dirt off from the bottom of the shoes. This is to prevent slipping. So you are encouraged to look at the hold before you step your feet on it.

Develop your foot strength first.

Experienced climbers have incredible foot strength. This is acquired over time and over countless practices, drills and actual climbs. As a beginner, you may not have as much foot strength yet. You need to develop it. Your choice of climbing shoes matters a lot.

While experienced climbers can get away with less-supportive shoes, you should stick to stiff soled ones as a beginner. Go for steady climbing. Do not rush the process. When you have finally developed or improved your foot strength for much more challenging climbs, you can probably go for less-supportive climbing shoes but understand that this will take time.

Master the footwork techniques.

There are plenty of ways to maximize the use of your feet during the climb. Among the most commonly used and easily learned techniques by beginners are edging and smearing. In this section, you will also learn more about other footwork concepts you may find useful in improving your rock climbing skills. You may not be able to master some of these techniques yet but you should at least realize that you can use your feet in more ways than you can imagine.

Edging

Edging is probably one of the most important things you need to master as a climber. You will find this footwork useful when you encounter smaller footholds. Small footholds do not allow your entire shoe to fit on it. This leaves you with two choices. These are to use either the inside or outside edge of your shoe.

The inside edge is the area of the shoe from the big toe down. The other edge is the area of the shoe from the pinky toe down. Edging is the technique used when you are focusing on either of the inside or outside edge of your climbing shoe in order to find your balance or to prepare for the next move on your ascent.

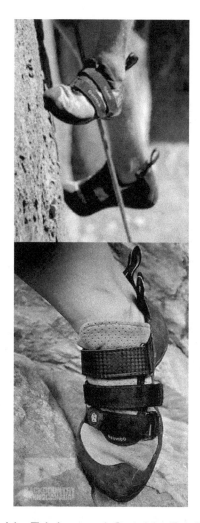

Inside Edging and Outside Edging

Now, which is best to use, inside or outside edge? Most climbers are more comfortable with using the inside edge. It is simply because the big toe has more power to push you up. There are cases however, when using the outside edge is more ideal.

For instance, if you need to move your body laterally along the rock surface, resting the outside edge of your climbing shoe on the foothold is best. Because the pinky is less nimble and generally weaker, it won't be able to hold your weight for long. In which case, you have to move much quicker when using the outside edge.

Climbing shoes in general, are decent enough for edging. However, the stiffer, flat-shaped kind is usually best for this footwork technique. That's because these kinds of climbing shoes are capable of absorbing more pressure and ease the stress on the feet caused by standing on a small foothold.

Smearing

So you think small footholds are a challenge? Where are you supposed to plant your feet when it looks like there are no available footholds at all? That's when the smearing technique comes to play.

Smearing is all about using the sole of the shoe against the slab or rock for support. It does sound scary when you think about it but what makes this technique work is friction. This is why you have to apply as much pressure to grind the sole into the rock in order to prevent your feet from slipping. It's as if you are squashing a bug. The amount of pressure required in smearing depends on how steep the terrain is.

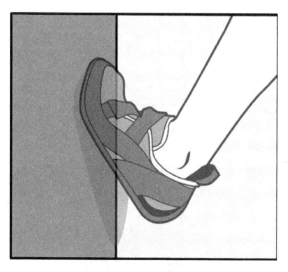

Image Source:
http://www.climbing.com/skills/training-7-simple-drills-to-improve-footwork-and-technique/

The best climbing shoe for smearing is the rubber kind. In this footwork technique, you will be relying on friction. In which case, you would want your shoes to have as much rubber as possible. Because the pressure will be applied on the toes, you are better off with flat shoes. Avoid the downturned type of climbing shoes.

Toe and Heel Hooking

For angled and steeper climbs, you need to apply more creativity. For such terrains, you need to treat your feet like they were your hands. In these situations, toe and heel hooking are the best options. Both give you the chance to take weight off from your hands and at the same time, help you prepare for the next tough move up.

In applying heel and toe hooking, pressure is essential. You need to apply as much pressure as you can against the rock especially if you are hooking for the next move.

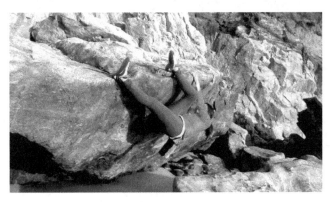

Image Source:
https://www.youtube.com/watch?v=T9bIIWK27F
A

Heel hooking is done by putting your heel on a foothold near your waist level and sometimes higher. The only difference with toe hooking is that you have to use your toes or the top of your foot instead. A heel hook is essential when you are climbing a roof, a ledge or an arête.

In this technique, you have to use the strength of your hamstring for pressure. You can do a heel hook on a jug, an edge or a knob. With this type of footwork, your arms and hands can be relieved on some of the weight so you can shake them off or rest them a bit until you are ready to make the next move. You can also use the heel hook to push your body up.

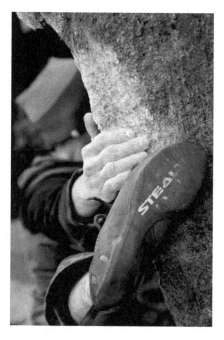

Image Source:
https://littlebangtheory.wordpress.com/tag/bould ering/

You can use toe hooking as an alternative to heel hooking. It works the same way except that pressure should be applied on top of the foot instead. A toe hook is helpful in keeping your body as close to the rock as possible.

Some climbing shoes are better for hooking than others. If you are more akin to heel hooking, it is best to choose a shoe with enough rubber around the heel. If you prefer toe hooking on the other hand, you should choose a shoe with better rubber toe patches.

Flagging

This technique is useful for preventing your body from swinging out and falling off. It involves the use of one leg pointed to a different direction than the rest of the body with the main objective of maintaining your balance. In other words, the extended leg is not used for support. Rather, it is merely for shifting the center of your balance. Take a good look at the images below.

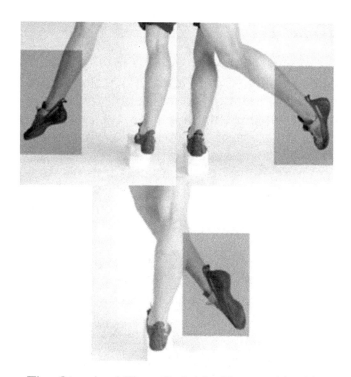

The Standard Flag, Outside Flag and Inside Flag

Image Source: http://www.climbing.com/skills/find-your-footing/

The other leg is extended either hanging or resting on a hold, the climber will lose balance. The standard flag is the easiest to learn and the first thing that beginners usually master.

Stemming

Have you ever done a split? It may be useful in rock climbing. This is a technique that requires the least amount of strength but it takes time to master. For this climbing technique to work, you must make use of the tension on your body to climb up as you push on holds. Climbers find stemming quite useful in dihedrals or inside corners. Stemming also provide a great opportunity for climbers to rest a bit and shake out their arms and hands.

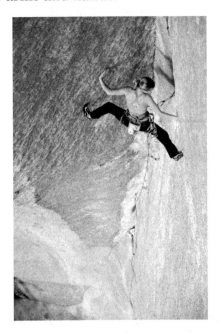

Image Source:
https://www.pinterest.com/farflungfitness/hiking-and-climbing/

Back Stepping

Beginners rely on a common step where they rotate their legs so their hips face the rock surface. If you learn to position one foot on a step so that the outside instead of the inside of your hip is facing the rock, your torso will be elongated allowing you to have a longer reach in that same direction while the other foot is in a flagging position to provide stability and balance. This is back stepping.

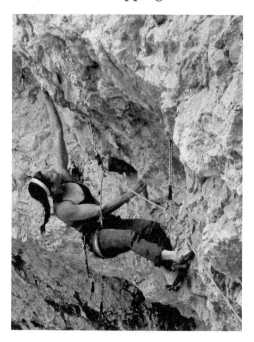

Image Source:
http://allirainey.com/home/2014/08/04/move-of-the-month-3-the-backstep-improve-your-climbing-series/

In this image, the climber has her left foot back stepping and her right foot flagging. This position allows her to reach higher with her left arm.

Do not let these techniques overwhelm you.

They look quite challenging. Most of them require flexibility. You will be able to master these techniques properly if you develop your flexibility first. So please take your time in practicing the movements along with some flexibility routine.

Chapter 3 – Get a Grip!

In addition to footwork, handhold techniques are also essential in rock climbing. Your hands and feet should be properly coordinated. Paying more attention to your feet should not mean completely ignoring your hands. They both need attention.

We dedicate this chapter for discussing the kinds of holds you may encounter, how you can grab them more effectively with proper handhold techniques and how you can improve your grip and overall strength. We'll start with a few tips.

Avoid over-gripping.

When the climb gets higher and steeper, it gets scarier. With fear comes a tendency to over grip. This causes a huge problem. Over-gripping quickly causes a vicious pump. It is difficult to recover from this. It drains strength. It makes a climber forget about technique. It makes a climber lose confidence.

Do not grip too hard on the hold. As much as possible, apply light grips. Remember, you have your feet to stabilize you. So you don't have to carry the weight on your shoulders.

Know which way to pull.

Pulling down comes naturally to us. It is similar to climbing a ladder. However, you cannot always apply a downward pull in rock climbing. In some cases, it is best to pull either sideways or upward.

Pulling to the side is preferable when you are climbing a steep rock with sideways orientation. By pulling to the side, you keep your weight on your feet and save upper body strength. An undercling or an upward pull on the other hand, is best when you have to reach for a faraway hold. It takes time to learn which way to pull but with practice, you will soon learn to do this by instinct.

Keep the arms straight.

When you're climbing a steep rock, avoid bending your elbows. Your arms should be kept straight. This prevents straining your biceps. By extending your arms, you are hanging from the bone instead which allows for better support. Bending your elbows however, may be unavoidable when it is time to crank a move. Make it quick though. You wouldn't want to deplete your biceps strength too much too soon.

Avoid overextending your arms.

In an effort to get a grip on a distant hold, there is a tendency to over-reach. Understand that your reach has a limit. Remember that you have a balance to maintain. You are working against gravity. When you make an attempt to reach too far, you may lose a grip on your feet which increases your chances of slipping. Instead of overextending your arms, try to move your feet upward. Moving your feet up first allows you to reach higher and farther with your arms.

Learn the best ways to deal with different types of grips.

There are various ways to grab on a rock. Just like with footholds, your grip should depend on the rock's orientation, shape and size.

Edges

These are probably the most common type of holds in rock climbing. They are a horizontally shaped handhold that comes with a positive outside edge. Some edges may also be rounded. There are flat edges but others are designed with a lip allowing climbers to pull out on them.

The sizes of edges vary. Some are thin and others are wide enough to accommodate the whole hand. Big edges are referred to as jug or bucket. Jugs are great for beginners who are yet to develop a strong grip. You will find them useful in climbing overhanging rocks. One of the basic ways to grab on edges is crimp grip.

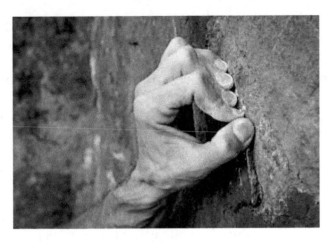

Crimping

Image Source:
http://anewdomain.net/2015/10/22/jason-dias-help-someone-just-wants-end/

Crimping provides a solid grip on the edge. The tips of your fingers are flat on the edge, arched above the tips. You have to be careful when using this type of grip. If you crimp too hard, you may cause damage on your finger tendons. When this happens, you will face some downtime. It may take months before you can recover from such an injury.

Slopers

These are rounded handholds which are common in slab climbs. Unlike edges, slopers do not come with a lip or positive edge where you can wrap the tips of your fingers around. Rather than relying on a solid grip, slopers require skin friction against the rock's surface.

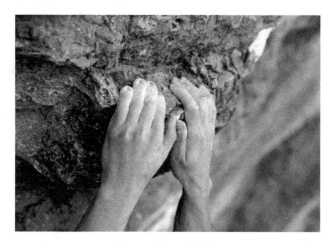

Open Hand Grip

Image Source:
http://breakingmuscle.com/strength-conditioning/the-3-types-of-grip-and-the-8-ways-to-train-them

Open hand grip is ideal for handholds with sloping edges. It is best to use this grip if you can count on skin-to-skin friction. While it may not be as solid as a crimp, the open hand grip can be just as strong especially with the help of a chalk. Friction increases with chalk on your fingers.

This type of grip takes some time to master. If you encounter this handhold, use your fingers to get a good feel around it. This will help you figure out the best part to grab on. Some slopers provide a bump or a slight ridge which allows climbers to apply a better grip. Once you have figured out the best part to hold onto, start wrapping your hand onto the handhold while keeping your fingers together. Use your thumb to press against a bump if the sloper has one.

Pinches

When edges protrude, they make crystals or small knobs on the rock surfaces. They are then called pinches. Most pinches are quite small and strenuous. The best way to grab them is through the pinch grip.

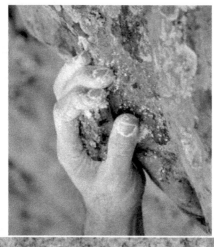

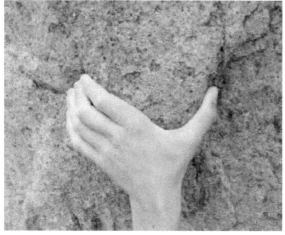

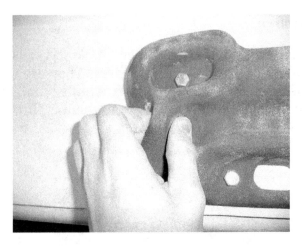

Pinch Grips depending on the size of the handhold

Image Sources:
http://climbing.about.com/od/RockClimbingTechniqu
e/tp/Nine-Basic-Types-Of-Climbing-Handholds.htm

http://www.climbingtechniques.org/intermediate-
moves.html

http://en-eva-lopez.blogspot.com/2013/02/training-
pinch-strength-for-climbing.html

Apply a pinch grip by literally pinching on the handhold with thumb on one side and the rest of your fingers on the other. Small pinches require your fingers and thumb to be close together. Stack your index and middle finger against the thumb. This will make the pinch grip much more solid.

Pockets

You may also encounter holes on the rock surface and you can use them as a handhold too. They are referred to as pockets. These holes come in various sizes and shapes. Some allow climbers to put as many as four fingers while others are so small, only one finger can fit into them. Some pockets are oblong shaped while others are flat. There are deep pockets and some shallow ones.

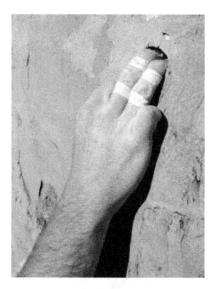

Image Source:
http://climbing.about.com/od/RockClimbingTech
nique/tp/Nine-Basic-Types-Of-Climbing-
Handholds.htm

When you do encounter pockets, assess it properly by inserting as many fingers as you comfortably can inside the hole. Get a feel inside. If you can feel lips or dimples inside the hole, use your finger tips to pull against them. If the pocket only allows one or two fingers inside, it is strongly recommended that you use your strongest fingers, either the middle or index finger or both if the pocket allows it.

Sidepulls

A diagonally or vertically oriented edge is referred to as sidepull. As the term itself suggests, this is a handhold located to your side and not above you. This handhold is meant to be pulled sideways rather than straight down. When you grab onto a sidepull, you need to counter the force of gravity by extending your other hand and feet to the other side.

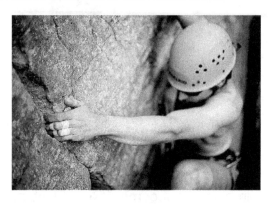

Image source:
https://www.flickr.com/photos/marc_robin/31683
5393

The opposing forces work in keeping your body balanced and stable. You can also turn your hip and lean it against the wall as you position the outside edge of your shoe on a foothold. While one hand extends on a sidepull in the opposite direction, you can now reach higher with the other hand.

Gastons

This type of handhold is similar to the sidepull as they are both diagonally or vertically oriented. However, while the sidepull is located to your side, the gaston is a handhold that you will find in front of you.

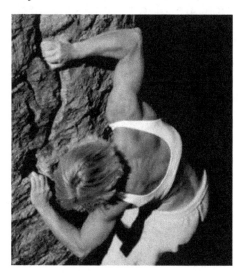

Image Source:
http://climbing.about.com/od/RockClimbingTech
nique/tp/Nine-Basic-Types-Of-Climbing-
Handholds.htm

You can grab this handhold using your fingers and palm as your thumb is pointed downward. Your elbows must be bent. Use your arms to pull outward as if you are trying to open a sliding door. This technique works best if your feet are positioned in a way that they oppose the pulling force of your hands. A gaston is a strenuous technique but you will find it useful in many routes. So take your time to practice and master the move.

Underclings

This handhold is grabbed on the underside. Use your fingers to grab the outside edge of the hold. These holds are of different sizes and shapes. They may come in the form of flakes, pockets, inverted edges, diagonal or horizontal cracks. Like gastons and sidepulls, these handholds demand body tension. Your hands and feet should be placed in opposite directions to strike a balance.

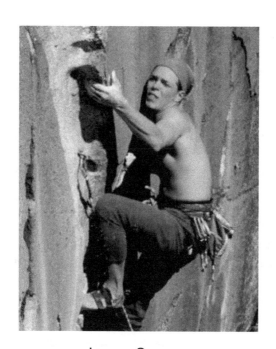

Grab the hold using the face of your palm up while your thumb points outward. Move up as you pull out the hold and plant your feet against the surface below in the opposite direction. You can also grab onto the hold with your thumb placed beneath it and your fingers on a pinching grip above.

These handholds work best if you grab them near your body's mid-section. The farther it is from your midsection, the more tension you will feel and the more chances you will lose balance. Because these holds are strenuous, it is advisable to straighten your arms. With your arms straight, your arms will suffer lesser muscle fatigue.

Palming

What if there are no handholds at all? Will you still be able to climb up then? When there are no holds to grab onto, you can use your palms instead. Use your open hand. The skin to rock friction with the heel of your palm against the rock surface will work to push your body up. This technique will also save you plenty of arm strength. Push with your palm instead of pulling your weight up with your arm and hand.

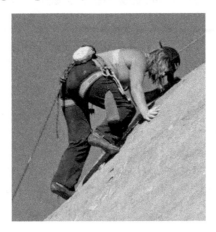

Image Source:
http://climbing.about.com/od/RockClimbingTech
nique/tp/Nine-Basic-Types-Of-Climbing-
Handholds.htm

Chances are the rock surface is not completely flat. You will find a dimple there. Place your palm toward the rock and press the heel on the rock. Your weight shifts from your foot to your palm. This will give you an opportunity to move your feet up. Remember though to keep your balance. Your other leg and arm should be placed in the opposite direction to make this work.

Matching Hands

This is simply about placing both hands on a hold next to each other. It is easier done on a wide edge. This handhold technique allows climbers to change hands so they can reach higher on a next hold. The challenge however, is when you are dealing with a rather small edge.

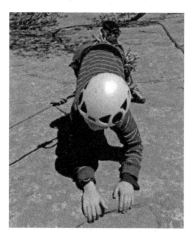

Image Source:
http://climbing.about.com/od/RockClimbingTechnique/tp/Nine-Basic-Types-Of-Climbing-Handholds.htm

Doing this technique is still possible but it is more difficult. In this case, match with your fingers instead of your whole hand. Start freeing one finger at a time on one hand so you can use it to reach for a higher handhold.

You need to strengthen both your feet and upper body to improve your climbing skills. You can practice these handhold techniques through indoor wall climbing. Some are more challenging to master than others. But over time, your body becomes more familiar with the moves until it is embedded in your muscle memory.

Chapter 4 – Learn Proper Body Positioning

So you've learned how to use your hands and feet, how to properly place them on the holds so you can climb more efficiently. But you need to learn one more thing about your most important tool, your body. To keep yourself balanced on the rock while spending the least amount of energy and effort, you also need to learn about proper body positioning.

Understand that there are various ways to place your hands, feet and body against the rock. Your main goal is to figure out the best way to position them in a way that you maintain your balance.

How to maintain balance?

We've talked about the importance of maintaining stability and balance. But what is it and how do you find it? The center of gravity in your body is found around your navel. You would want to keep this point at the center in between the various points of contact on the wall. By being aware of your center, you are better off finding the best ways to position your body so that most of your weight rests on your feet rather than your arms and hands.

While you may have a strong upper body, your forearms are not designed to carry all the weight.

In fact, this is the weakest link. Your legs are stronger which is why you need to be more conscious about them and maximize their use.

When you are climbing, you place yourself in a constant battle against gravity. You cannot eliminate gravity. It will pull you down if you let it. You are given an important tool however. You can use your entire body to work around this obstacle.

So now, we will take a look at proper body positioning according to a rock's orientation. Remember, you have to work with gravity. Working against it is futile so pay attention.

How to position your body on vertical walls?

On a vertical wall, your feet are perpendicular to the ground. You can get most of your weight on your feet by positioning your body as close to the wall as possible. You can do this by moving your hips near the wall.

When you pull your hips away from the wall, you can notice that the weight shifts from your feet to your arms. This is not preferable because by doing so, you put yourself at work against gravity. What you ultimately want is to work with gravity. Keep your hips close. Be mindful of this as you make your ascend and at each and every step up just like the climber does on the image below.

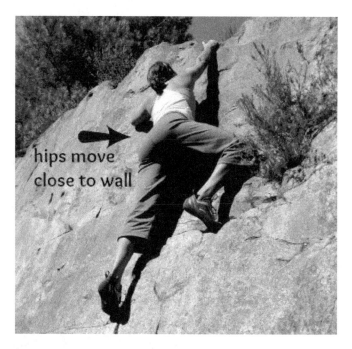

hips move
close to wall

Image Source: http://conquerthecrux.com/rock-climbing-basics-part-1-efficient-body-positioning/

How to position your body on a slab?

The pull of gravity is straight down when your body is perpendicular to the ground. As the rock surface's orientation changes, it is important that your body positioning is adjusted accordingly. On a slab for instance, you will encounter small handholds. It will require you to use smearing technique. In this case, your feet is already taking much of the weight and your arms are their only for support and balance.

While keeping your hips as close to the wall as possible works on a vertical wall, this body positioning is not ideal on a slab. This is one of the many mistakes climbers make. Do not allow yourself to be caught in the same pitfall.

Take a good look at the image below.

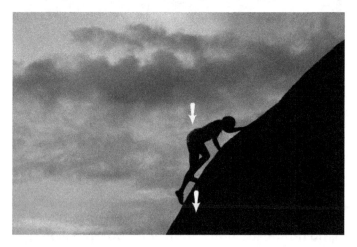

Image Source: http://conquerthecrux.com/rock-climbing-basics-part-1-efficient-body-positioning/

The climber is pulled down by gravity at 90 degrees. In which case, positioning her body at 90 degrees is the most efficient way of making the climb. Why? With her hips away from the wall, her feet take majority of her weight. In this position, she allows her bottom half to push straight down as she works her way up with her arms and moves her feet along with it.

This body position also maximizes the surface area covered by her feet on the slab. It gives her feet more friction which is critical in smearing. In other words, by positioning her body this way, she works with gravity by allowing gravity to pull her onto the wall.

How to position your body on an overhang?

Overhangs are a tricky bunch. With this kind of rock orientation, you need to expect your arms to take more weight. This is where you need to put your upper body strength at work. It doesn't mean however, that all your weight should be carried by your arms. There is still a way to lessen the tension and avoid working against the pull of gravity. Let's use this image as reference.

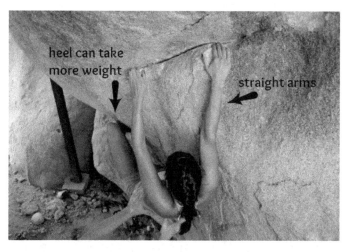

Image Source: http://conquerthecrux.com/rock-climbing-basics-part-1-efficient-body-positioning/

Notice that the arms of the climber are hanging off from the hold. Her hips are close to the rock and she doesn't let her feet hang. She keeps them glued on a foothold. Can you guess what will happen if she bends her elbows or lets her hips sag or her feet hanging? She will fall quickly.

Bending the elbows will only increase the tension in the area which can only take so much strain. If she lets her hips move away from the wall, she loses her feet's hold as well. She will slip off. In this scenario, a heel hook works best.

There is more to this though. To conquer an overhang, a climber needs more than upper body strength. It requires core strength as well as good technique. And it requires a lot of time for practice.

Warm up properly.

When you are up on the wall on a tough climb, you will have a harder time being conscious about your body positioning. This is why it is important to keep practicing proper body positioning during warm up.

You can always rely on strength to make the ascent but there is always a smarter way of making the climb. You can make the ascent with much more ease. You can make it less strenuous. The more you give time for practice and warm up, the more it becomes second nature to you. Moreover, core strength is essential in climbing too. It will be helpful for you to incorporate some core strengthening exercises for your warm up.

Chapter 5 – 10 Rock Climbing Essentials

Rock climbing is not a cheap hobby. But the exhilarating feeling of climbing is priceless. Now you can make do with your buddy's spare shoes and share equipments. But if you are serious about this, you have to invest more on your improvement. Improvement includes buying the essential equipments.

Climbing Shoes

Your feet are essential tools and you can maximize their usefulness during a climb with the right kind of shoes. Climbing shoes are made of sticky rubber soles. This design allows climbers to make the most of friction. They are flexible and supportive enough to help you strengthen and protect your feet at the same time.

Choose climbing shoes that fit tightly. They are to be worn without socks. There are 3 different styles of climbing shoes you need to know about. These are slip-on, Velcro and lace-up. If you enjoy long climbs, the lace-up shoes are best because they aren't easily taken off. If you prefer quick climbs such as bouldering and sport climbing however, the two other styles are ideal.

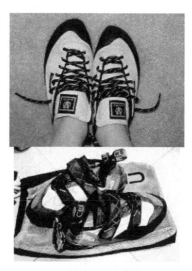

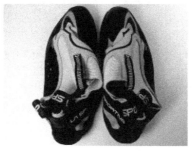

Climbing Shoes: Lace-Up, Velcro and Slip-On

Image Sources:
https://www.flickr.com/photos/38220692@N03/3525651544/

https://www.flickr.com/photos/39559809@N05/7935863452/

https://www.flickr.com/photos/supertopo/5635602613/

Your climbing shoe requirements can change. As a beginner, you have to choose one that is comfortable to wear around. At this stage, you are to focus on easier climbs. No complex foot placements yet. As you move one level after another, you may need to upgrade to a climbing shoe that is more tightly fit. Shoes with down-turned toes are extremely uncomfortable but they are very much useful for climbers who are attempting to conquer technically difficult routes.

Chalk

Another climbing essential you should not forget about is chalk. Climbing chalk is made of magnesium carbonate. The same kind used by gymnasts. You need chalk to protect your hands from rubbing and chafing against the hard rock surface. You also need it for a better grip on the handholds.

Climbing chalk comes in different forms. While loose chalk is convenient, block chalks are much cheaper. Chalk balls are also available. You can use them by simply shaking them onto your fingers. Choose according to your preference.

Chalk Bag

If you have chalk, you need a bag to put it into. There is nothing technical about this climbing essential. As with chalk, you can choose one that you are most comfortable with as long as the bag is equipped with a solid waist belt and a reliable buckle. Its opening at the top should comfortably accommodate your hand as you reach for some chalk.

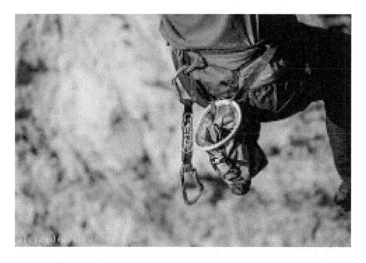

Image Source:
https://www.flickr.com/photos/alex_ito/97302562
51/

Carabiners

Often referred to as "biners", these are metal loops designed with a gate where webbing and rope can pass through. The gate can be closed shut creating a more secure closed loop. Carabiners used to be made from steel but the modern kind is made using high-grade aluminum.

There are various kinds to choose from. Some are designed with key-lock gates while others have wire gates. Because the rope is least likely to be caught on its nose, the key-lock kind is an excellent choice. Inspect the carabiners before you buy them. Look for signs of wear and tear. Most importantly, you should test and make sure that the gate opens and closes in a smooth manner.

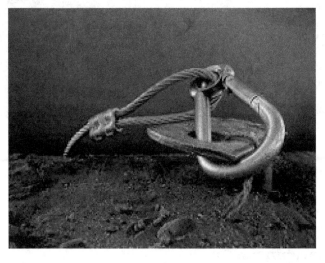

Image Source:
https://www.flickr.com/photos/die_ani/10235172/

Locking Carabiners

The difference between locking carabiner and the normal carabiner is that the former are designed with locking gate and a cover. This is extremely important for all climbers. It is an essential ingredient to complete your belay device and it will complete a top-rope system. Inspect the equipment well before paying for it. For your sake, you may want to choose one that can work well under different conditions.

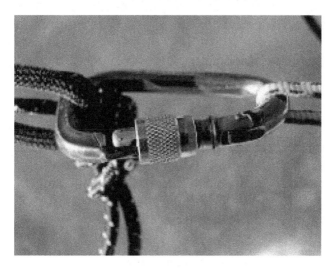

Image Source:
https://www.flickr.com/photos/24946690@N03/5
601126516/

Harness

Harnesses for climbing are made from a durable system that consists of webbing loops. It wraps around the waist and legs for optimum support. A harness is equipped with metal buckles for attachment. It also has a loop meant for attaching the belay device. You can also use it for carrying gear.

A harness is incredibly thin and lightweight but it is amazingly strong and sturdy. Because a harness is one of the most essential equipments that complete the climbing safety system, it is extremely important for you to invest in an excellent quality one. Do not skimp on a harness.

It is strongly recommended that you buy a new one. And while you are at the store, give it a test ride. While comfort is not a concern in climbing shoes, it is for harnesses. Remember, you will be wearing it most of the time during your climbing spree and you should be comfortable and supported enough by your harness.

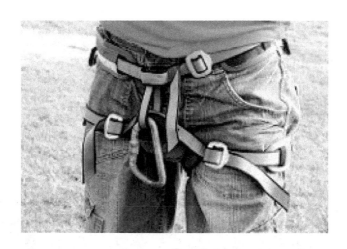

It may also be smarter to choose one with four gear loops on its belt. It is not necessary for top-roping but if you ever decide to upgrade to trad and sport climbing, you will need it. Paying some extra now will save you the trouble of buying another one later. The cost of climbing harnesses varies but a good quality one may start at $60.

Belay Device

The climber and the belayer work together. The belay device is attached to the belayer's harness which it allows the belayer to control the rope's movement. As the belayer locks the device off, the rope is prevented from escaping. This is essential to the safety of the climber. The belay device can stop a devastating fall.

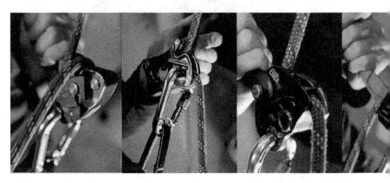

Belay Devices

Image Source:
https://www.flickr.com/photos/55080027@N07/5475184599/

Modern belay devices are made from aluminum. They attach to the belayer's device through a carabiner. There are many kinds and brands to choose from. The simplest kind is the Black Diamond ATC. Mammut, Trango, Metolius and Black Diamond ATC are designed with teeth which makes it quite easy to lock. Among the most excellent auto-locking belay devices in the market are Trango Cinch and Petzl Grigri 2.

Dynamic Rope

As a climber, this is your lifeline. Dynamic ropes are made from polymers that are highly engineered to stretch into thinner fibers. They are composed of two parts: the kern and the mantle. The kern is the rope's core made from long, elastic and strong fibers. The mantle on the other hand, is wrapped around the core that serves to protect it and at the same time make it easier to handle.

Because it's too important, there are plenty of things you need to consider when buying a dynamic rope. First, you have to think about the length and diameter. The standard rope length is 50 meters. However, this may be too short for rappels and sport routes. To be on the safe side, you would want to get a longer one. 60 meters may be enough especially if you are only planning on buying one.

Second, you have to consider if you want the more expensive dry treated kind. A dynamic rope that is not dry treated is likely to deteriorate easier with exposure to water and moisture. It also proves difficult to use under wet conditions. With a dry treated rope, you won't have these problems. The catch is that the dry treated kind is much more expensive.

Third, you have to think about the diameter. The recommended rope diameter depends on the kind of climbing you prefer. For instance, a dynamic rope with 8.9 to 9.4mm in diameter is excellent for long trad climbs. On the other hand, a rope with 9.5 to 10.5 mm in diameter is best for traditional and sport climbing as well as top-roping.

Thicker diameter ropes are heavier and may be more difficult to handle through the belay devices. Thinner ropes are lighter and much easier to handle. The problem is they are less safe.

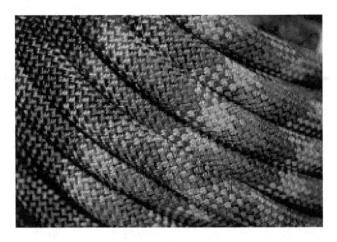

Image Source:
https://www.flickr.com/photos/dualshotty23/4886
969504/

An excellent quality dynamic rope may cost you a minimum of $120. As with harnesses, avoid buying used ropes. Also, you have to constantly expect your rope for damages. Ideally, they should last for 3 years before they are to be replaced but if the rope show signs of serious wear, it needs to go.

Quick Draws

This is simply a combination of two carabiners combined together by what is referred to as a dogbone. This dogbone prevents the carabiners from rotating. Quick draws are quite useful for attaching to bolts and for building a top-rope anchor.

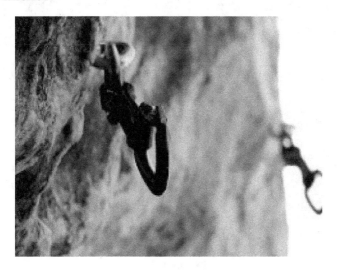

Image Source:
https://www.flickr.com/photos/97603845@N00/2
209133156/

Webbing

This is essential for anchoring the top-rope system. Trees and boulders may be used as anchors. The webbing is what you use for these anchors. Unlike a dynamic rope, webbing is not as expensive. You can get it at different lengths. For starters, you may want to invest in webbing with 17-, 26- and 51-foot sections.

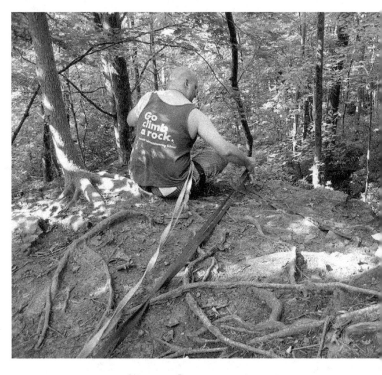

Image Source:
https://www.flickr.com/photos/anotherpintplease/
320118764/

Chapter 6 – Anchoring, Knotting and Belaying

So you now know how to move your feet, hands and body. You understand how to choose your equipments. Now, we will delve into how to make use of these equipments for your safety.

Understanding the Basic Principles of a Standard Anchor

The entire climbing safety system depends on the anchor. That's how important this is. This is also why you are strongly advised to consult a professional about it. This section is only meant to help you understand the basic principles and does not suffice as a main guide.

There are a few basic things that you need to look for and make sure of before setting up an anchor. And these principles include the following.

Use SOLID ANCHORS only.

As mentioned before, you can use a tree or a boulder as an anchor. It has to be solid and steady. Never rely on an anchor that may snap easily like a dead twig. You need to find sturdy points of connection. This is also why you need extra webbing so you can set up a sturdy anchor even if it means something farther away.

REDUNDANCY is essential.

Always think of backing up your anchor. You need to have a minimum of two points of connection. If one fails, you still can count on another.

EQUALIZE your anchors.

If you're using two anchors, you have to make sure that the load is shared between them equally. This will assure that a fall can be held and your weight is supported as you lower.

NO EXTENSION allowed.

A slack in the connecting points is dangerous to the climber as it also increases the strain to the anchor. We will talk about minimizing extensions later using the right kind of knots.

Watch out for SMALL ANGLES.

Ideally, the angle should not exceed 60 degrees. You should keep it at a 20 degree angle. Wider angles can create bigger amount of force which you wouldn't want to happen.

To make sure you remember these basic guidelines, think **SARENE-SA**.

Use **S**olid **A**nchors

Make it **R**edundant

Make sure it's **E**qualized

Allow **N**o **E**xtension

Use **S**mall **A**ngles

This acronym may save your life or another's!

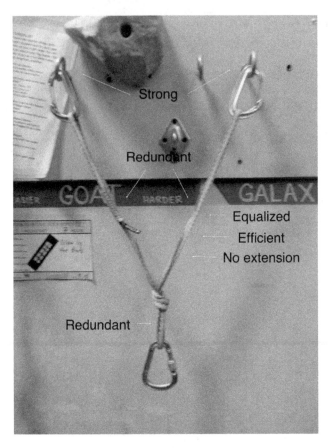

Strong

Redundant

Equalized
Efficient
No extension

Redundant

Image Source:
https://www.pinterest.com/robbthorn/climb-on/

The image below is an example of how the belay system is set up. In this case, one solid anchor is used, a tree.

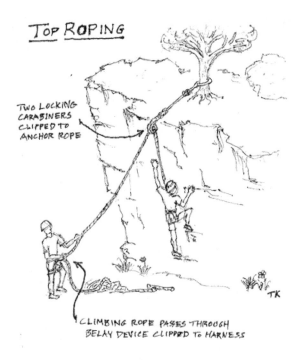

TOP ROPING

TWO LOCKING
CARABINERS
CLIPPED TO
ANCHOR ROPE

TK

CLIMBING ROPE PASSES THROUGH
BELAY DEVICE CLIPPED TO HARNESS

Image Source:
http://www.alpineinstitute.com/articles/expert-tips/rock-climbing-terms-styles-and-techniques/

Understanding Basic Knots

We will discuss four basic knots here and their applications. This should be enough for a beginner to get started.

Figure 8

One of the easiest to tie and the strongest, the Figure 8 can be used to attach into the harness.

It can also be used to attach another closed loop to a tree trunk. Follow the image below for a step-by-step procedure for tying the knot.

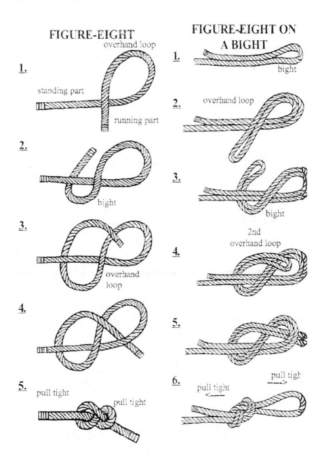

How to make a Figure 8 knot on a Bight

The Figure 8 in a bight is ideal because you are most likely to use a carabiner for attachment; you need the hole to make that possible. Do not forget to pull as tightly as you can.

Girth Hitch

This knot is most useful in setting up anchors especially if you're using a natural anchor. It is also best for connecting two loops together. The best thing about the Girth Hitch is that they are quick and easy to make. It also causes less strain on the rope or webbing.

The image below shows you how to make this easy knot.

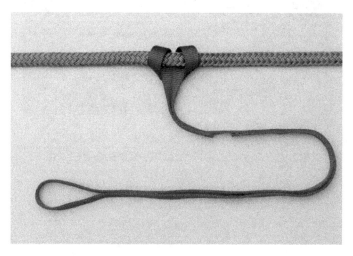

Image Source:
http://www.animatedknots.com/girth/#ScrollPoint

It is important that you hitch using the most stable and thinnest part of the object. In the example below, the part right above the root of the tree is ideal. Why is this important? If you tie it up at the thickest part, it is likely to slip to the thinner areas when it is pulled tightly. But if you have it on the thinnest part, there is lesser likelihood of it slipping and that means a more stable climb and also safer for the webbing.

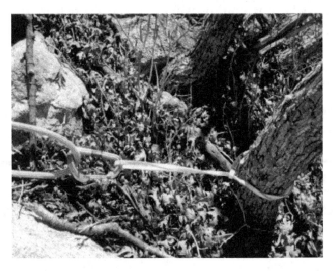

Image Source:
http://www.climbingtechniques.org/girth-hitch.html

Clove Hitch

Like the Girth Hitch, the Clove Hitch is also useful for building anchors. You can use this knot to attach an object to the rope center as well as attach yourself through your harness to an anchor. Another application of the Clove Hitch is for making a carabiner block that makes a single-rope rappel. This is best used by climbers though for securing themselves as they reach the top of a climb in place of a personal anchor.

This is how you make a Clove Hitch.

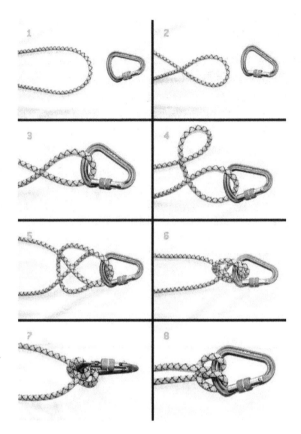

How to make a Clove Hitch

Image Source:
http://backcountryskiingcanada.com/forums/view
/general-talk/top-six-climbing-knots-you-need-to-
know

Munter Hitch

This is one of the most versatile knots and it's pretty basic too. Most climbers rely on this knot for rappelling purposes. It can also be used as a back-up system so climbers can stay safe on a long climb in case they drop their belay device.

In some cases, the Munter Hitch may also be used as a replacement for a belay device although this is not advisable. Using the rope for this purpose may be safe for the climber but not for the rope as it will only cause serious damage and lead to unnecessary rope wear.

You can refer to the image below for making a Munter Hitch.

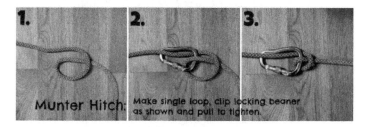

How to make a Munter Hitch

Image Source: http://conquerthecrux.com/8-essential-climbing-knots/

And this is how you can secure a Munter Hitch.

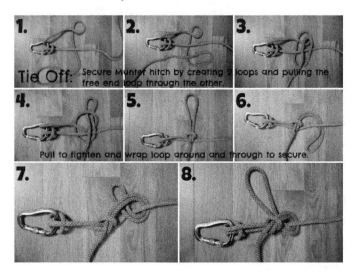

How to secure a Munter Hitch

Image Source: Image Source:
http://conquerthecrux.com/8-essential-climbing-knots/

For now, you can make use of these knots for your needs. As you climb more often and immerse yourself deeper or higher into the rock climbing world, you will be able to pick up more ways to knot your rope.

Understanding Belaying Basics

Belaying is one of the first things you need to master before you even place a hand on the rock. To be a good climber, you need to be a good belayer first. As a belayer, the safety of the climber becomes your responsibility. We call the rope the climber's lifeline because in case the climber falls, his weight shifts from the rock to the rope. Your role as a belayer is to break that fall. You can do so by providing a break on the rope.

It is also your responsibility to ensure that everything from the knots to the harness and the entire belay system is properly in place. Do not forget to check on your harness and that of your climber.

In this section, you will learn how to give a top rope belay.

Set up the belay.

The first thing you need to do is to set up the belay device. The manner of feeding the dynamic rope into the belay device varies from one brand to another. Follow the instructions on the manual. Once the rope is fed into the belay device, attach the locking carabiner through the loop and the rope. Next, attach your harness to the locking carabiner and lock it. Make sure everything is securely locked.

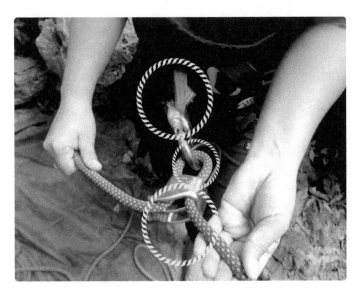

How to prepare the belay

Take the athletic stance.

Remember that as a belayer, you are providing support for your climber. Put your legs apart at a shoulder width distance. Make sure your body is well balanced and your feet are stable and firmly planted on the ground.

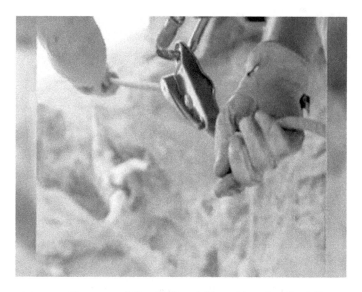

Image Source: http://allonhill.net/rock-climbing-basics-toprope-belay-technique/

Stand where you can see your climber and the route he/she is taking. It will be helpful if you take your place close to the rock. By keeping close to the rock surface, you reduce the distance essential in case of a fall.

Choose which hand to use for the brake.

The dominant hand should be used to provide a brake and the other hand serves as guide. Refer to the image below for proper hand positioning on the rope.

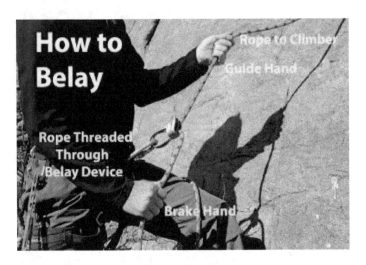

How to Belay

Rope to Climber

Guide Hand

Rope Threaded Through /Belay Device

Brake Hand

Image Source:
http://climbing.about.com/od/learninghowtobelay
/a/LearntoBelay.htm

Your hands should stay on the rope at all times as you keep an eye on the climber. The illustration below shows you how to take in the slack from the rope as the climber ascends to the top.

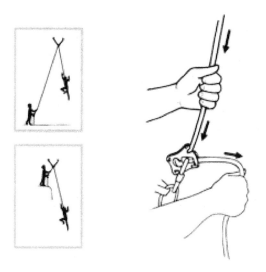

Image Source:
http://www.mountaineeringmethodology.com/bel
ay-device-click-up/

Pull on the rope with your guide hand. Without taking the brake hand off the rope pull on the rope away from your hips. Make sure this hand is ready to brake at all times.

When the climber is ready to come down, follow the instructions below, images 4 to 6. You need to create a slack now so your climber can come down. Feed the rope into the belay device from your brake hand to the guide hand. To make sure the climber has a smooth landing, break the feed from time to time.

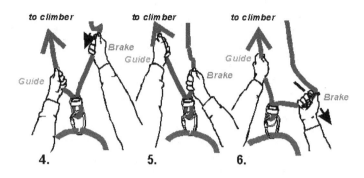

Image Source:
https://www.princeton.edu/~oa/climb/belaywal.sh
tml

Go over the safety commands.

With the climber and the belayer a couple of feet apart from each other, a simple script should be followed to ease understanding and communication. The safety script goes like this.

Climber: "ON BELAY?"

The climber asks the belayer whether or not everything in the belay system is securely attached.

Belayer: "BELAY ON."

The belayer assure the climber that the belay system is ready and that he/she is prepared to brake the rope in case of any falling accident.

Climber: "CLIMBING."

The climber is ready for take-off. He/she puts his/her life on the hands of the belayer now.

Belayer: "CLIMB ON."

The belayer gives the climber the thumbs up.

When the climber is ready to come down, he/she should shout out the word, "DOWN." The belayer ensures the rope is tight without any slack. The belayer will then instruct the climber to take his/her hands off the rock surface. Then the belayer guides the rope so the climber can start rappelling.

Chapter 7 - Strengthen the Climbing Warrior Within

"You will climb only as high as your mind lets you." ~ Robyn Erbesfield

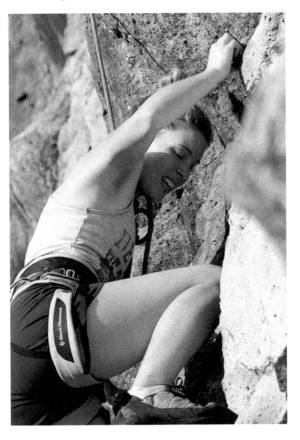

Image Source:
https://www.flickr.com/photos/grahamcamero
nhimself/9757722134/

Climbing isn't just about strength and stamina. It is not just about movement. It is definitely physically challenging. But it is as much as a mental challenge as it is physical.

Without the right mindset, the right attitude, the drive to make the next move, the passion to keep going and the confidence to finish, physical strength matters a little less. When you are facing a steep climb, you need focus. You need to remain calm and relaxed. You need to clear your mind so you can concentrate on the task at hand. This won't happen if you do not have a climbing warrior mindset.

Strength of the mind is just as important as the strength of the body. So we take this time to focus on improving the quality of your thinking.

Do not tie your self-image to your performance.

This has been the downfall of many. Of course, it is heartbreaking to have to work hard, to spend your time and energy only to fail to achieve the results you expected. But you have to accept the fact that you or anyone for that matter, cannot do everything perfectly every time. And you don't have to. Your best is enough.

Your achievements do not define your worth as a person. Detach your self-image from your performance. Focus on the process of learning and of improving rather than on the outcome. This will not only reduce the greatest cause of frustration. It will also help you enjoy climbing as it should be first and foremost, enjoyed.

Free yourself from the ties that bind your perception of self value to your chosen sport. It is liberating. It reduces anxiety and pressure. When you are free from these negative thoughts and emotions, you will climb more freely. You will climb better. You can climb more happily!

Surround yourself with positivity.

Negativity is draining. It is mentally, emotionally and physically straining. Remember that our thoughts and actions affect that of other people. The thoughts and actions of other people also affect us. If you are climbing with equally frustrated people who complain about everything, you are likely to carry the same burden of negativity. The downward pull of this negative energy is stronger than the pull of gravity.

What you need instead is positive aura. Choose your climbing buddies well. Surround yourself with upbeat, positive and motivating people. Positive energy is just as contagious as the negative kind. It will allow you a huge deal of enjoyment. And the gift of their motivating words and attitude can also make a huge impact in the improvement of your skills and technique.

Be ready to leave your comfort zone.

In climbing, it means reaching as far as you can even if it causes you some physical discomfort. It means pushing your body to endure more. And you can absolutely endure more if you are mentally ready. Being mentally ready means pushing your fears aside and considering what seems to be impossible, possible!

Just because you are used to be on this level of thinking does not necessarily mean it's good for you. Sometimes, all you need to do is to entertain the idea that you can do much more, that you are capable of bigger things to make it into reality.

Assess, understand and manage the risks.

Stretching the limits of your comfort zone does not mean banishing your fears altogether. A healthy amount of fear is good. It makes you cautious but not overly cautious. It prevents you from taking unnecessary risks.

You have to understand that pushing your body to do more is coupled with risks. In a feat as dangerous as climbing, you have to be realistic without being negative. You have to set proper expectations without limiting your own capabilities. You have to learn to be objective.

Understand the risks involved. When you understand them, you are more capable of making the situation less risky. You can have safety precautions in place. The key here is preparedness.

Build your confidence.

Self-confidence is tied to self-image. If your self-image suffers, your confidence plummets with it. Negative thoughts about poor performance along with negative words like "I don't," and "can't" will cause your confidence to suffer.

Take a 180 degree turn. Put the past where it belongs. Put it behind you after you have taken the valuable lessons. Take the valuable lessons and use them for self improvement. What did I do wrong during that climb? What technique should I have used to get a better outcome? How do I improve this specific technique so I can do much better next time?

Focus on the things that you can control. That's your improvement. Concentrate on the things that you can do. Avoid obsessing about what could have been that does not translate to anything productive.

Use visualization.

Instead of obsessing about past mistakes and poor performances, why don't you go back to the things that you did right. Try to visualize and re-live those moments over and over when you're feeling the negative vibe creeping in. Re-living these great events, the exhilarating feeling, the rush of happiness and excitement flowing through your body creates a positive ball of energy that you can use to pick yourself up from your past frustrations.

Celebrate your victories no matter how small they may seem. They are a testament that you are doing some things right. This is the moment you allow your confidence to be lifted. More confidence goes a long, long way in your future endeavors.

Love climbing unconditionally.

Do not love climbing for the outcome. Love it despite all the cuts and bruises, the frustrations, the hardships, the sweat and tears. Happiness comes to those who love unconditionally, without expectations, without conditions, without barriers and borders. Love freely. Climb happily!

Conclusion

Thank you again for purchasing this book!

I hope this book was able to help you learn the basic techniques and skills you need to get started on climbing. It is up to you now to take all the things you've learned here and put it into good use.

Happy climbing!

CPSIA information can be obtained
at www.ICGtesting.com
Printed in the USA
FSHW02n2307010518
47696FS